Cancer Guided Imagery Program

for
Radiation, Chemotherapy, Surgery
and Recovery

Steve Murray CHt.

First Printing

Body & Mind Productions

Cancer Guided Imagery Program
for
Radiation, Chemotherapy, Surgery
and Recovery

Published by
Body & Mind Productions
820 Bow Creek Lane Las Vegas, NV 89134
Website: www.cancerimagery.com
Email: bodymindheal@aol.com

First Printing November 2003

Library of Congress Cataloging-in-Publication Data
Murray, Steve
Cancer Guided Imagery Program for Radiation, Chemotherapy, Surgery and Recovery
/ Murray, Steve – 1st ed.
Library of Congress Control Number 2003107849
ISBN # 0-9742569-0-0
Includes bibliographical references and index.
1. Cancer 2. Cancer Guided Imagery 3. Guided Imagery
4. Imagery 5. Visualization 6. Self-Healing 7. Psychotherapy

Cover design: Jay Trujillo
Type design and production: Gracie Garcia
Editor: Stacey Abbott

Printed in U.S.A.

VIDEOS-DVDS-BOOKS

By
Steve Murray

VIDEOS & DVDS

Preparing Mentally & Emotionally
For Cancer Surgery
A Guided Imagery Program

Preparing Mentally & Emotionally
For Cancer Chemotherapy
A Guided Imagery Program

Preparing Mentally & Emotionally
For Cancer Radiation
A Guided Imagery Program

Preparing Mentally & Emotionally
For Cancer Recovery
A Guided Imagery Program

Dissolving & Destroying Cancer Cells
A Guided Imagery Program

Pain Relief Subliminal Program
Let Your Unconscious Mind Do It!

Fear & Stress Relief Subliminal
Program Let Your Unconscious
Mind Do The Work!

30-Day Subliminal Weight Loss
Program Let Your Unconscious
Mind Do The Work!

30-Day Subliminal Stop Smoking
Program Let Your Unconscious
Mind Do The Work!

BOOKS

Cancer Guided Imagery Program
For Radiation, Chemotherapy, Surgery,
And Recovery

Stop Eating Junk!
5 Minutes A Day-21 Day
Program

The Reiki Ultimate Guide
Learn Sacred Symbols and Attunements
Plus Reiki Secrets You Should Know

3

DISCLAIMER

The only people who may claim to cure cancer are Medical Doctors. The publisher and author are not Medical Doctors. It is important to understand that Relaxation and Guided Imagery cannot cure cancer. They are to be used in conjunction with medical treatment prescribed by Medical Doctors. This book makes no claims that Cancer Guided Imagery can cure cancer. This book is sold with the understanding and intent that the publishers and author are not engaged in giving medical advice in this book. It is recommended you seek professional medical treatment for cancer. It is advised to check with your doctor before starting a Cancer Guided Imagery Program.

DEDICATION

To My
Mother and Father

FOREWARD

When faced with a disease like cancer, I feel the best thing to do is to open your mind up to all the possibilities available, of course with common sense. Combining competent medical care with the power of your mind in a positive manner is by far the best combination for health and well-being. I should know.

A very invasive breast cancer tumor of 2.5cm was suddenly discovered in me. It terrified me tremendously and I immediately started doing Cancer Guided Imagery while I worked with my doctor. In less than a month the tumor ended up measuring only 1.2cm and was totally contained at the time of my surgery. No need for radiation or chemo. I was extremely happy and pleased, and I know Cancer Guided Imagery helped me in preparing for my successful treatment and recovery.

I suggest you at least try the program presented in this book for 60 days. I believe that if you combine Cancer Guided Imagery with your medical treatment you will have positive results.

To your health,
Leticia M. Oliver, DCH, CSC

INTRODUCTION

I understand that a person in the beginning of a cancer challenge is usually overwhelmed and time is of the essence. Because of that, I strove to write a clear-cut, easy to read and understand book on Cancer Guided Imagery. I feel that I have accomplished that. With this book you are able to get a quick overview of how and why Cancer Guided Imagery is successful, and then step-by step instructions so you can start your Cancer Guided Imagery Program right away. If you have any questions, please feel free to contact me at bodymindheal@aol.com.

Steve Murray CHt.

SPECIAL THANKS

To M.D. Anderson Cancer Center at the University of Texas for being the first to have my Cancer Guided Imagery Programs available for patients on their video on demand system.

———

CONTENTS

"Make your own recovery the first priority in your life."

-Robin Norwood

Chapter One

What is Guided Imagery?

The ability and power of the mind to help influence the body in healing is quite extraordinary, and at times, it seems unbelievable what can transpire with this powerful influence. This book presents information and guidance for applying a proven process called Guided Imagery, which will help you tap into this powerful influence for cancer treatment and recovery.

Guided Imagery has been called the language of the mind. It is a language that the mind can use to talk to the body, a language the body can understand immediately and without question. It is a way of communicating internally with the parts of ourselves that cannot speak in words.

Guided Imagery is an internal process that creates *messages* with images–which will be fully explained later. These *messages* include directions and goals that are communicated to your entire body and/or any area you choose. For this reason Guided Imagery has been labeled a "mind intervention with the body." This intervention incorporates the power and resources of the mind to convey the positive responses and changes you desire.

Guided Imagery has also been described as the interface, or connection between the body and the mind because of the positive chemical and biological changes it can produce in the body. These changes are extremely useful in the successful treatment of and recovery from cancer.

Internal and External Images

The mind processes images, consciously and unconsciously, throughout all aspects of life and then communicates them to the body. The sources of these images can be external, outside the body or internal, inside the mind.

We are all familiar with the language of internal images in our dream experiences, both day and night. When the mind recalls events from the past, or contemplates about the present or future, it uses internal imagery. The sparkle of the sun on the ocean, a loved one's face, the sound of church bells, the aroma and flavor of our favorite foods and the anticipated events of a future vacation if created in the mind, are all examples of internal imagery. External images are gathered by our five senses as the events and circumstances take place outside the body and are then processed through our mind. These external images give us information for how our body should respond. If you are standing in the middle of the street and you hear, see, maybe even feel a speeding car, your mind will process these external images. The body will first receive a message and react chemically with a burst of adrenaline. Secondly, the body reacts physically to the message, and you quickly move your body out of harm's way.

The difference between Guided Imagery, dreams and other internal imagery, is that Guided Imagery intentionally creates imagery inside the mind that has directions and goals for the desired present and future. Other internal images are usually not intentionally created and therefore they generally do not have desired directions or goals.

It is important to note that all external and internal images are processed by the mind; consciously and unconsciously, then communicated to the body.

Guided Imagery

Guided Imagery is a flow of imagery or images that you create internally which consists of thoughts that have directions and goals. The dictionary defines *thought* as: *the act or product of thinking*. The dictionary defines *think* as: *to form a mental concept of: imagine*. So your thoughts can form mental concepts that are created internally from your imagination. Imagination will be discussed in a later chapter and you will discover how it plays a vital role in Guided Imagery.

These thoughts (mental concepts) can be one or a combination of sounds, feelings, smells, visuals, and tastes, which can represent the desired present and/or future.

21

Essentially, all your thoughts become internal images and they have a direct influence on your body. Of course thoughts can either be positive or negative. Guided Imagery uses only positive thoughts.

The body can perceive Guided Imagery as reality and will respond as if it has truly experienced, or will experience the perceived imagery. The body can respond to real (external) events the same as imagined (internal) events. This phenomenon will be fully explained in chapter three.

There is no known harm that Guided Imagery can cause when used with positive intentions. It is a very personalized and unique process because it develops differently in each individual. The Guided Imagery that is highly effective for one individual may not be as effective for someone else. Because Guided Imagery is entirely internally driven, each person can decide when, where and how it is used. The great news is that anyone can learn to do it and have positive results.

Guided Imagery and Healing

Guided Imagery has been used as a healing tool by most cultures and civilizations throughout history. It has been and still is a very important part of many religions, old and new. Navajo Indians still practice an elaborate form of Guided Imagery that encourages a person to see him or herself as healthy and strong. Ancient Greeks such as Aristotle and Hypocrites believed that images released spirits in the brain, which stimulated the heart and other parts of the body. They also believed that the strong image of a disease was enough to cause its symptoms, which is a belief that many people still hold today.

It is a well-documented occurrence that some medical students will experience symptoms of the diseases they are studying at that particular time. Hypochondriacs are also known for experiencing many symptoms of many diseases. If the mind can manifest symptoms in the body, it follows that the mind can also make symptoms disappear.[1]

In ancient Egypt and during Biblical times, Guided Imagery was essential to the medical treatment of physical ailments. Historically, Western Medicine has largely ignored the mind when treating diseases of the physical body.

In the past, Doctors generally administered the recommended medical treatment available to treat only the body. The mind was seldom ever considered in any of the prescribed treatments. Now however, the current medical community of the Western world is becoming increasingly aware of the affect that personal attitudes and beliefs have on the treatment and recovery of the body from illness and disease.[2] It has started to acknowledge the mind-body connection as a very important factor in healing and recovery.

Research findings continue to establish Guided Imagery as an effective process for improving health.[3] A growing body of medical research shows that Guided Imagery can have a

---

[1] See Selected Bibliography
[2] See Research and Reference
[3] See Research and Reference

powerful influence on every major control system of the body. [4] It can stimulate vital functions like heart rate, blood pressure, local blood flow, wound healing and even the immune system. This of course, is vitally important to the treatment of, and recovery from cancer.

In many instances even *ten minutes* of Guided Imagery can reduce blood pressure, lower cholesterol and glucose levels in the blood, and heighten short-term immune cell activity. It can considerably reduce blood loss during surgery and reduce the amount of morphine needed after the procedure. Furthermore, Guided Imagery can reduce headaches and pain and has been shown in numerous instances to reduce the adverse effects of chemotherapy; especially nausea, depression, and fatigue.

Guided Imagery and Visualization

A common misconception is that Guided Imagery is the same as Visualization. It is not. Visualization is a technique that only requires pictures in the mind, without the other elements described earlier such as sounds, feelings, smells, tastes or a combination of them.

The challenge with Visualization is that some people cannot see and/or experience pictures in their mind. Guided Imagery is not Visualization, although Visualization can be a part of Guided Imagery. It was explained earlier that the definition of *think* is *to form a mental concept of:*

---

[4] See Research and Reference

imagine. Mental concepts are the main component of Guided Imagery. For the purposes of this book we will say that a mental concept is made internally, inside the mind, and can consist of one, all, or any combination of the following elements: sounds, visuals, thoughts, touch, feelings, inner sensations and smell. Basically anything that can be created or recreated in your mind is done with mental concepts. Do not panic if you can only use or create one or a few of the elements described in a mental concept. The more sessions you do with Guided Imagery, the more elements you will be able to incorporate into your mental concepts. Remember, everyone is unique; and develops his or her mental concepts differently. Also, keep in mind that there is no correct or incorrect combination of the elements in your mental concepts.

To reiterate, Guided Imagery consists of more than just seeing visual pictures in your mind as in Visualization. However, if you can see pictures in your mind it can be a part of your Guided Imagery. Remember, many individuals are unable to see pictures in their minds, but they can still do Guided Imagery very effectively.

Guided Imagery, Self-hypnosis and Meditation

Guided Imagery incorporates some components of meditation and self-hypnosis. Like meditation, with Guided Imagery you get in a relaxed state. But with meditation your goal is to get into a deeper relaxed state. With most meditations you are asked to "let go of all thoughts, and clear your mind." During Guided Imagery, however your goal is to get into a relaxed state, but not as deep. You do not want to let go of your thoughts, just the opposite; you want to have certain thoughts you created with directions and goals. Like meditation, self-hypnosis is also done in a relaxed, but deeper state usually called a trance. It is accomplished most of the time by giving yourself only verbal or silent suggestions for what you want to happen and/or change. For example; when a person is in a deep trance and suggests to him or herself that they will be calm and confident when applying for a job, qualifies as self-hypnosis. But, in a focused relaxed state you imagine applying for the job with all or some of the elements mentioned before (visuals, sounds, feelings etc.) and then imagine getting the job. That is Guided Imagery.

You do not have to believe in Guided Imagery for it to work. You just have to have an open mind each time you do it. Many people who were initially skeptical and/or challenged by Guided Imagery were able to achieve outstanding results as their sessions progressed. The Guided Imagery they really had doubts about, or thought was not strong enough to produce positive results, did. One's skill level improves with each session, thereby enhancing the positive results of Guided Imagery.

"The best and most efficient pharmacy is within your own system."

-Robert C. Peale

"The wish for healing has always been half of health."

-Lucius Ammaeus Seneca

Chapter Two

Cancer Guided Imagery

Cancer Guided Imagery is Guided Imagery that is focused on Cancer Treatment and Recovery. The imagery includes directions and goals for *preparing* mentally and emotionally for cancer treatment, having *successful* cancer treatments, and having a *successful* recovery.

Cancer Guided Imagery is now being used in support groups and hospitals throughout the country with several different variations and techniques.[5] None of these variations and techniques are wrong, because *they all will work*. It's just that there are different degrees of difficulty in learning and doing them. This book was born out of the need for a simple-to-understand and effective "step-by-step" book on Cancer

---

[5] See Research and Reference

Guided Imagery that incorporates the best of the various techniques used by cancer support groups and hospitals.

I feel the Cancer Guided Imagery techniques presented in this book are the most effective, simple, and easy to learn. And they will enable you to start using Cancer Guided Imagery for your own cancer treatment and recovery right away.

These techniques should be thought of as complementary healing and recovery tools to be used with traditional medical treatment. They are tools that will help improve your chances of success in the treatment of and recovery from cancer.

There are many important factors that come into play for successful cancer treatment and recovery—your medical doctor, nurses, hospital staff, relatives, friends, and support groups all have a powerful impact. The choice of cancer treatment, drugs, and therapy are also important parts of treatment and recovery. The most vital part of successful treatment and recovery from cancer is YOU. Cancer Guided Imagery is one method that can help strengthen the role the patient plays in achieving success with cancer treatment and recovery.

Research and Cancer Guided Imagery

There have been many tests, research studies, and books written in the last 20 years about Cancer Guided Imagery, the importance of personal beliefs, positive attitudes and the role the mind plays in the successful treatment and recovery of cancer patients. [6]

The Simonton's were pioneers in the field of Cancer Guided Imagery and the body-mind connection. Their best-selling book, <u>Getting Well Again</u> was published in 1979. [7] They established one of the first protocols for Cancer Guided Imagery. This was considered a breakthrough event in a field that had plenty of anecdotal information, but very little scientific proof.

Since the Simonton's book was published, additional research has been conducted with cancer patients, using Cancer Guided Imagery and Relaxation Techniques during their treatment and recovery. [8] This research shows that both processes produced positive results. It was determined that Guided Imagery, when used in conjunction with a Relaxation Technique—which will be discussed in detail in later chapters—produced better results for patients in their treatment of and recovery from cancer.

Studies have also found two important facts regarding cancer patients. Having a positive outlook on cancer treatment and recovery as a patient, combined with having a high confidence level with their doctor, produced better results with cancer treatment and recovery. [9]

Again, research has shown Cancer Guided Imagery will

---

[6] See Research and Reference
[7] See Selected Bibliography
[8] See Research and Reference
[9] See Research and Reference

31

help instill and reinforce a positive outlook and confidence in your doctor and treatment.

Cancer Guided Imagery Will Help To:

➢ Prepare the patient mentally and emotionally for any kind of cancer treatment.

➢ Obtain knowledge about cancer treatment and recovery, which will enable educated adjustments or changes regarding the ideas, beliefs, and interpretations pertaining to cancer treatments and recovery.

➢ Empower the patient to actively participate in treatment, recovery and the entire healing process. When you actively participate in regaining your health, it automatically boosts confidence and optimism.

➢ Reduce any feelings of hopelessness and helplessness. You will feel more in control and better able to cope with these feelings.

➢ Decrease any tension and stress throughout the body, which will provide a sense of peace and tranquility that may never have been experienced before.

➢ Release any negative thoughts and beliefs about cancer treatment and recovery.

➢ Reduce overall fear, which can become overwhelming at times. Having cancer can create many real and imagined fears.

➢ Tap into inner strengths and find hope, courage, patience, perseverance, love and other qualities that will help with your cancer treatment and recovery.

➢ Reduce the level of discomfort during cancer treatment and side effects after the treatment.

➢ Keep positive attitudes and expectations during treatment. This will increase the chances of a successful recovery.

Cancer Guided Imagery Caveats

There have been claims of healing from cancer using Cancer Guided Imagery alone. **This book does not encourage this practice**. Patients should always follow their doctor's advice regarding the prescribed medical treatment and recovery program. As explained earlier, Cancer Guided Imagery is a program that should be used in conjunction with your prescribed medical treatment and recovery program. Cancer Guided Imagery is *not* about instant healing, it is a process, a self-help program. Some results may happen immediately, other results may need several weeks or longer for sessions to produce any noticeable effects. Patience and perseverance are also necessary components of Cancer Guided Imagery. Healing and recovery can and should happen on many levels. With any illness, you may experience emotional, mental or spiritual healing before any physical healing occurs. Eventually there should be healing and change on all levels for long-term cancer recovery.

"The miracle of self-healing occurs when the inner patient yields to the inner physician."

-Vernon Howard

"We are what we think. All that we are rises with our thoughts. With our thoughts we make the world."

-Buddha

Chapter Three

How and Why Cancer Guided Imagery Works

The main reason Cancer Guided Imagery is very effective is that the physical body can react to images created internally in the same way as it reacts to images created externally. Many responses in the body cannot distinguish between an image experienced externally—happening outside the body, then processed by the mind, and an image experienced internally—created inside the mind. The goal of Cancer Guided Imagery is to create new, positive internal images of the desired present and future, and communicate them to your body.

As explained in chapter one, the difference between external and internal images lies in the source of these images. External images come from outside the body and are based on whatever is happening at the time. They originate and are created from your five senses: smell, sound, taste, touch, and sight, which are processed through the mind and are then communicated to the body. Internal images used in Cancer Guided Imagery are created mentally from memories, experiences, thoughts, emotions, intent and imagination, which will then be processed through the mind and communicated to the body.

An example of external imagery could be a happy family gathering or any happy meeting with friends. The senses are constantly taking in the information from your surroundings while you are at this gathering, and are then processed by the mind to your body. Your body then responds to these images by getting into a happy, warm, content, loving state; a condition conducive to healing. This is experiencing external imagery.

Now, if you go into a quiet room and imagine the gathering before it happens with similar details, the mind would process this internal imagery to the body. You could elicit the same response from the body as with external imagery if you were actually at this type of event. This is experiencing internal imagery.

Here's another example of how external and internal images affect the body. When a person is in an actual suspenseful or dangerous situation, external images are created through the senses, then processed through the mind and communicated to the body. The body then responds with a fight-or-flight response, which releases adrenaline throughout the body. The body is then ready for action; a confrontation or a retreat to safety. Again, when one goes to a quiet room and imagines a suspenseful or worrisome situation using Guided Imagery, the mind will process this and will react with an identical fight-or-flight response. In actuality there is no danger, but the body's chemistry reacts as if it were in a dangerous or suspenseful situation.

Imagination

The dictionary defines *imagination* as: *the act or power of forming mental images of something not present to the senses or not previously known or experienced.* The imagination is also the source of creativity and problem solving abilities. All these qualities of the imagination are needed, and used in Cancer Guided Imagery sessions.

Imagination is another prevailing reason why Cancer Guided Imagery is so very effective and powerful. When doing a Cancer Guided Imagery session you are focusing and directing the imagination. It is the imagination that allows the creation of the desired present and future into mental concepts, which is a very important ingredient in Cancer Guided Imagery.

Aristotle said the imagination was "the window to the soul." Einstein stated, "Imagination is more important than knowledge." This book upholds a similar message:

the imagination, when used properly will become one of a person's greatest assets for cancer treatment and recovery.

The Placebo Effect: Imagination at Work

Imagination is what drives Cancer Guided Imagery. Imagination can provide a powerful source of healing to the body. The link between imagination and healing in patients has been studied in Western Medicine, and it has been named "The Placebo Effect" or it is also known as "positive expectant faith."

The Placebo Effect is a common occurrence in the patient who has pain relief and physical healing even though an actual treatment is not given.

The Placebo Effect is created when the patient is told by the doctor to expect certain results from a specified treatment and/or therapy he or she is given, but the treatment or therapy is not actually performed. For example a patient may be given sugar pills instead of actual medication. The patient believes and imagines the results that he or she is told to expect, either consciously, unconsciously or both. The body then responds to the imagination and manifests the results that the patient was told to expect, thereby activating "The Placebo Effect."

The Placebo Effect has been shown in many scientific

studies to be responsible for 35 to 55 percent of the effectiveness of all treatments, including medicine and surgery. It is important to point out even though the imagination is used in the Placebo Effect; it is not focused or guided as it is in Cancer Guided Imagery. This might be the reason why people get varying results from the Placebo Effect and why it doesn't work for everybody.

Cancer Guided Imagery produces higher percentages of positive results because the imagination is focused, and it has directions and goals, which are reinforced during sessions.

A Placebo Effect

In 1962, a surgical procedure was developed to improve blood flow to the heart for people suffering from major heart disease. The operation relieved patient's pain 80 percent of the time, and improved the ability of the heart to pump blood throughout the body by 70 percent. A documented scientific study of the Placebo Effect was then performed at Johns Hopkins Medical Center in conjunction with this surgical procedure. Two groups were brought together of the same age, sex, and the same level of heart disease. The heart surgery was done on one group, and not the other (placebo) group. The placebo group had the identical surgical incision, but no actual surgery to the heart. The results were dramatic! The two groups had *identical success rates* in both pain relief and enhancement of their heart function. The placebo group imagined (because they thought it was performed) the successful surgery and the body responded to their imagination.

This study and similar studies are convincing demonstrations of the power of the imagination. It is clear that the imagination can be an important and powerful force when used in Cancer Guided Imagery.[10]

---

[10] See Research and Reference

"The natural healing force within each one of us is the greatest force in getting well."

-Hypocrites

"It's the repetition of affirmations that leads to belief. And once that belief becomes a deep conviction, things begin to happen."

-Claude M. Bristol

Chapter Four

Imagery Content

Imagery Content is used for every Imagery Suggestion during a Cancer Guided Imagery session. Without Imagery Content, you cannot perform a Cancer Guided Imagery session. Imagery Content is also very personalized for every individual. This chapter is about how to acquire Imagery Content.

As one progresses through cancer treatment and recovery, his or her Imagery Content will need to adapt to changing needs and circumstances; although some of the Imagery Content might remain the same throughout all your Cancer Guided Imagery sessions. Changing Imagery Content will depend on what is personally needed at any given time during cancer treatment and recovery. Before we go on to learn how to acquire Imagery Content consciously and unconsciously, let's first define and explain an Imagery Suggestion.

Imagery Suggestion

An Imagery Suggestion, which can also be a statement, always includes a direction or goal that the patient wants to manifest during cancer treatments and recovery. One or a group of Imagery Suggestions make up a Cancer Guided Imagery Session. Again, what is used for the suggestion is the Imagery Content.

At the end of this book there are chapters of Cancer Guided Imagery sessions, which provide proven suggestions for you to use. The Imagery Content for these suggestions however are highly personalized and must be acquired on an individual basis as is detailed in this chapter. You can do one, or as many of the suggestions that you have time for in any one session.

Once you become accomplished at performing Cancer Guided Imagery, the Imagery Content for a suggestion should only take two to three minutes to complete. That is plenty of time to communicate it to the body. Of course for some people it may take longer. If that is the case you might want to cut back on the suggestions during a session. Of course, suggestions should be carried out at one's own pace. Eventually, if you can do it in two to three minutes, wonderful! If it takes longer, do not worry; a suggestion can be effective regardless of the pace at which it is performed.

The suggestions outlined in the Cancer Guided Imagery sessions in the chapters at the end of this book are ideal to start with. Many patients may find that these really are the only ones they will ever need. If, however other circumstances arise which require different suggestions, one can certainly make his or her own. Regardless of their source, there are a few basic elements the suggestions should contain. They have to have directions, goals, and/or desired outcomes, and be in a logical sequence.

For example you would use the following suggestions in a logical sequence during a session: "I imagine myself prepared mentally for my Chemotherapy treatment." Followed by, "I imagine myself peaceful and calm during my Chemotherapy treatment," then "I imagine my cancer cells being dissolved and destroyed during my Chemotherapy treatment." You would not do "I imagine my cancer cells being dissolved and destroyed during my Chemotherapy treatment," then "I imagine myself prepared mentally for my Chemotherapy treatment." Now if you are only performing two suggestions in a session and for example they are, "I imagine my cancer cells being dissolved and destroyed during my Chemotherapy treatment," and then "I imagine my remaining cells healthy throughout my body" of course you would do the dissolving suggestion first. When you decide what and how many suggestions you are going to use, take the time and put them in a logical sequence before the session. The suggestions for the sessions in this book are already listed in the right sequence.

Whether you decide to create your own Imagery Suggestions or use the Imagery Suggestions in this book, the Imagery Content is still acquired the same way.

Acquiring Imagery Content

Once an Imagery Suggestion has been decided upon, for instance, "I imagine myself prepared mentally for my Chemotherapy treatment," you can acquire the Imagery Content in different ways; consciously, unconsciously, or both.

Consciously acquiring Imagery Content simply means being awake and aware when acquiring, planning and researching the Imagery Content for a suggestion. This Imagery Content can be derived from what you personally feel needs to change, happen, or be achieved. It can also be from medical advice, friends, support groups, books, published articles, and/or other valid sources.

Unconsciously acquiring Imagery Content for a suggestion is done in a relaxed state during sessions or even from dreams. This Imagery Content comes from the unconscious mind and usually is very powerful and timely.

Let's take the suggestion, "I imagine myself prepared mentally for my Chemotherapy treatment" and demonstrate how to acquire the Imagery Content for it both ways; consciously and unconsciously.

Consciously Acquiring Imagery Content

First, you should research all the information possible regarding mental preparation for Chemotherapy that you feel pertains to you personally. This information can be from doctors, appropriate material from books and articles, the web, support groups and other suitable sources. Talking to other patients who have mentally prepared for Chemotherapy successfully can also be beneficial. Find out from these patients what has and has not worked for them. Talking with other patients who have successfully been through treatment and recovery will be one of the most important resources in gathering conscious Imagery Content.

Select only the information that feels comfortable and resonates well with you. Separate this information into individual segments and write each one down. Then take a look at each segment and number them in an order you feel would be the most helpful, the first segment being the most important. The list of segments will now be your choices for the Imagery Content of this suggestion. Usually this list will provide at least a few, if not many selections of Imagery Content. Only one selection for a suggestion should be used during each session. Start with number one, then as you do other sessions, you can change the selections when and if you feel the need.

Acquiring conscious Imagery Content for suggestions is always an on-going process. The list can grow throughout the progression of your treatment and recovery. For instance: during a support group meeting, you learn what another woman has done to prepare herself mentally for Chemotherapy treatment. That information may feel right to you as well. Hence, it is added to your Imagery Content list for the suggestion, "I imagine myself prepared mentally for Chemotherapy," for use in a future session.

Usually the majority of Imagery Content you will have comes from acquiring it consciously.

Unconsciously Acquiring Imagery Content

Another option for obtaining Imagery Content is from the unconscious mind. It is a very easy process to do, but unfortunately for some people it does not always work during every session. It is undeniable however, that the more one uses this process the more successful he or she will be in getting Imagery Content this way. You will likely discover that Imagery Content acquired unconsciously is very powerful and pertinent.

Before a session begins, decide you are going to acquire your Imagery Content unconsciously. You have your suggestions for this session selected beforehand and they can be listed on paper, recorded on an audiotape or can be memorized.

You do the Relaxation Technique (explained in the next chapter) and then state your first suggestion on your list either out loud or silently. Do this even if you have the suggestion recorded or memorized. Then wait for any information, directions, guidance, or goals to float up from the unconscious mind that relate to the suggestion. This should only take five to ten seconds, and you do not have to think about it, just let it happen. Once the Imagery Content is received for the suggestion, perform your Guided

Imagery with it. When that suggestion is completed, the same process is done again for the next suggestion, and so on. Always use the Imagery Content that comes up first for the suggestion stated, do not wait for other content.

Example

State the following suggestion out loud or silently, "I imagine myself prepared emotionally for my Chemotherapy treatment." After it is stated, what floats up is that fear has recently become stronger upon entering the Chemotherapy room and during treatment. What also comes up is the need to be calm and peaceful before and during the treatment to neutralize the fear. With the information you acquired, the Imagery Content would be imagining yourself before and during the next Chemotherapy treatment being calm, peaceful, and without fear. You would imagine that and then repeat the same process with the next suggestion.

If Nothing Floats Up

If you are acquiring Imagery Content unconsciously, and after the suggestion is stated, nothing floats up to your mind related to the suggestion within 30 to 60 seconds, the suggestion can be turned into an Affirmation. How to turn a suggestion into an Affirmation and then what to do, will be explained in detail later on in the chapter. After the Affirmation, you go to the next suggestion. The same process gets repeated: state the suggestion, and use what first floats up for your Imagery

Content. Then if the same thing occurs—nothing floats up—do the Affirmation, and move to the next suggestion and so forth.

When you have suggestions that were turned into Affirmations during a session, you have several options. You can try again during the next session to acquire the Imagery Content unconsciously. You can be prepared for the next session with Imagery Content acquired consciously for the suggestions. Or you can try acquiring the Imagery Content from your dreams.

Imagery Content from Dreams

Another way to acquire Imagery Content from the unconscious mind is from dreams. Imagery Content from dreams is very effective and creative. There are people who use this method and it works so well for them, they use it the majority of the time.

At first with this method you might have sporadic or no results. Do not get discouraged and stop trying to obtain Imagery Content this way. Just keep practicing it and you will be successful.

The Process for Dreams

When acquiring Imagery Content from dreams, I recommend only working on one suggestion at a time. Although some people can receive content for more than one suggestion on any given night, one suggestion per night is ideal. Working on one suggestion at a time provides more quality and effective Imagery Content from dreams.

Once again, everybody is different when it comes to the whole process of Cancer Guided Imagery. So, if you would like to try and acquire Imagery Content for more than one suggestion in a night, do it. You will likely learn that this process works more effectively during different periods of time than others. This is why it is so important to be persistent with this method. If it does not work one week, try the next. Otherwise, you might be losing access to valuable Imagery Content.

Steps

The steps to obtaining Imagery Content from dreams are as follows: before going to bed at night, write down the suggestion(s) that need Imagery Content. Read the suggestion(s) out loud or silently before going to sleep. You may awake in the middle of the night from a dream with the Imagery Content for the suggestion(s), or the content may be there in the morning when you wake up.

Sometimes, although the content was received during a dream, you may have no memory of it in the morning. During the day, however, it is common for memories of a dream to surface at the conscious mind. When that happens just write the Imagery Content down. Of course, it is always possible that you might not receive any Imagery Content at all during the night. If this happens, just try another night.

It is a good idea to keep a pen and paper available next to the bed in the event that Imagery Content is received in the middle of the night or in the morning. Always write down any Imagery Content immediately, whether it is received in the night, morning or throughout the day.

Use All Three Ways

It is helpful to try and use all three ways to find out which is the most effective for obtaining Imagery Content. Feel free to do the method that proves to be the most fruitful. The way you acquire Imagery Content can be changed from session to session. You will discover one method produces better results than another at different times. The key is to be flexible and open to using all three methods. You might want to try a combination of methods during a session. For example, you have acquired Imagery Content for half the suggestions consciously before a session and you acquire Imagery Content unconsciously for the remainder of the suggestions during the session.

Affirmations

I am sure you have heard one of the most famous Affirmations made over a hundred years ago by a man named Emile Coue (1857-1926), "Every day in every way I'm getting better and better."[11] Affirmations are positive statements that usually reflect the present tense of a desired state of a person—physically, mentally, spiritually, and emotionally, or a combination of a few. These statements are repeated

---

[11] See Selected Bibliography

over and over again, silently or out loud for a certain period of time. Repeating these statements focuses the conscious mind on the desired state and helps the unconscious mind manifest this state. Affirmations can influence both levels of the mind, conscious and unconscious.

Affirmations are very powerful and they do work. There are many books written on Affirmations and much research done on the positive effects Affirmations can have on a person. I have listed a few at the end of the book.

Affirmations are incorporated into Cancer Guided Imagery in two ways.

The first method is when one is attempting to acquire Imagery Content unconsciously for a suggestion, and nothing floats up from the unconscious mind. The suggestion can then be turned into an Affirmation. The Affirmation should be repeated for several minutes silently or out loud, then you move on to the next suggestion.

The second alternative, because of time constraints and/or circumstances you are prevented from doing a full Cancer Guided Imagery session, you can just do Affirmations. The Affirmations should be about your cancer treatment and recovery. Just do as many as you can. This will maintain the continuity of your on-going Cancer Guided Imagery sessions.

The Cancer Guided Imagery sessions in the chapters at the end of this book provide Affirmations with the suggestions. This will make it easy to have Affirmations available for both instances. Following a few simple directions can also create cancer treatment and recovery Affirmations.

Creating Your Own Affirmations

There are a few simple guidelines to follow when creating one's own Affirmations for cancer treatment and recovery. Affirmations are stated in the present tense, and are personal and positive. They usually start with "I." An effective Affirmation needs to be specific enough to have a clear, conscious meaning for you. Positive Affirmations can also be used to release any negative ideas and beliefs concerning cancer and recovery.

Let's use the example suggestion: "I imagine myself prepared mentally for my Chemotherapy treatment." The Affirmation would be the following: "I am prepared mentally for my Chemotherapy treatment."

Repetition is one of the main reasons why Affirmations work. By repeating them over and over, they are instilled into the conscious and unconscious mind to make the statements become a reality. Only Affirmations which are appropriate for you should be used. The words that form the statement must feel comfortable. You can include words in an Affirmation that have a special meaning for you, but they have to be in the present tense. As you progress through cancer treatment and recovery, Affirmations might need to be adjusted in accordance with your changing needs and circumstances.

Affirmations can also be written down, taped, or memorized. They can be said out loud or silently. Affirmations can be repeated as many times as you feel is necessary or time allows. As a basic guideline, each Affirmation should be repeated for a minimum of two to three minutes. Generally, ten is the maximum number of Affirmations that can be effectively completed during any one session.

It is helpful to keep a running list of Affirmations while adding new ones. This way, you can choose the appropriate Affirmations when you need them.

"The power of imagination makes us infinite."

-John Muir

Chapter Five

Relaxation and Cancer Guided Imagery

As was previously stated, studies and research indicate that Cancer Guided Imagery works best when it is used in conjunction with a Relaxation Technique. It was found that Cancer Guided Imagery is most effective when the person is in a relaxed, but focused state of consciousness. This state can be induced by a Relaxation Technique, which then enables the Imagery Content to be processed and travel more easily from the mind to the body. Relaxation is very essential for Cancer Guided Imagery to be successful.

Relaxation techniques have been used in many forms of meditation by many cultures for thousands of years. One of the pioneers of Relaxation Techniques is Herbert Benson M.D., who published a best-selling book, The Relaxation Response. [12] This book explains in detail the benefits that

---

[12] See Selected Bibliography

relaxation has on the physical body and mind. It also includes medical and scientific research and studies to support these ideas.

When the physical body is relaxed, it becomes highly receptive and open to Cancer Guided Imagery. Once the body is relaxed the mind soon follows. The Cancer Guided Imagery you create in this state is more effective and produces positive, stronger results. Also when the body and mind are in a relaxed state, brain waves are lowered. This helps to release brain chemicals that act as natural tranquilizers for the body. These natural chemicals then lower blood pressure, heart rate, and anxiety levels. Research concludes that the whole body chemistry changes into a healing mode and helps to stimulate the immune system when it is in a relaxed state.

Research also suggests that some of the positive physiological impacts of relaxation may be the result of its effect on slowing the excess release of the hormone, Cortisol.[13]

Cortisol

The release of Cortisol is helpful during the fight-or-flight response and usually is triggered by fear and/or stress. Cortisol release is needed for the body to cope and survive those circumstances; however the release of Cortisol is intended to last for only a brief period of time. A continual, prolonged release of Cortisol,

---

[13] See Research and Reference

that can be caused by on-going fear and stress from cancer will inhibit the immune system and even cause tissue damage in the body. Relaxation aids in the regulation of this hormone by putting the body and mind in a peaceful, non-fearful state.

Relaxation Technique

There are many different Relaxation Techniques that work well when performed properly. You should always do one at the beginning of every Cancer Guided Imagery session. The Relaxation Technique I present in this book is a combination of a few well-known techniques. It was designed to ease you into a state of relaxation — not to induce sleep--but to shift the body, and then the mind into a relaxed state quickly. This will put you into a perfect state for a successful Cancer Guided Imagery session. Once you become accustomed to doing the Relaxation Technique at the beginning of each session, you will find yourself slipping into this relaxed state quicker each time you do it.

Most people find they have increased and/or renewed physical energy and a state of well-being as they incorporate relaxation into their Cancer Guided Imagery.

Relaxation is simply a process of letting go, and it is easy to learn and do with practice. The following are the directions and script for the Relaxation Technique to be performed at the beginning of your Cancer Guided Imagery session. This is the one I like and recommend, but feel free to use another Relaxation Technique if you prefer. Just make sure you do one before your session.

Directions for Relaxation

➤ Have the relaxation script ready for your session. You can write it down, use the book or record the script. After a period of time, you should be able to do it from memory.

➤ Maintain a passive attitude, do not strain, but enjoy the experience of the body as it relaxes and lets go of all tension and stress.

➤ If distracting thoughts occur with your relaxation session, gently replace them with the current relaxation direction. With practice distracting thoughts will come less frequently to the mind.

➤ Before starting the relaxation script, take five to ten deep breaths. When you exhale on each breath, say out loud or think the word "relax."

➤ After the five to ten breaths, just breathe at a normal pace and stop thinking or saying the word relax when you exhale. You then start the Relaxation Technique.

➤ When doing the relaxation script, state each body part direction out loud or silently before you do it.

➤ Allow at least 60 seconds to do each body part direction. Additional time can be spent relaxing a body part if you feel the need.

➤ After the whole body is relaxed, you are ready for a Cancer Guided Imagery session.

Methods for Relaxation

There are two methods for doing the Relaxation Technique presented here, and both are very effective. Try each one, and then continue with the method that works the best for you.

First method – Say each body part direction silently or out loud before you relax it. You then focus on the part and imagine it relaxing with all the stress and tension leaving it. This is done for at least 60 seconds. Then you continue to do each body part in the script the same way.

Second method – Say each body part direction silently or out loud before you relax it. Then tense it for 20 to 30 seconds. Next, release the tension and relax it for at least another 20 to 30 seconds, feeling the tension and stress leaving it. Then continue to do each body part in the script the same way.

As I mentioned earlier, more time can be spent relaxing any body part. But, after a little bit of experience with this Relaxation Technique, the recommend time of 60 seconds for each body part is generally sufficient.

The following is the Relaxation Script. Make sure you do the five to ten deep breaths with the relax command before you start.

Relaxation Script

- I now relax and let go of any tension and stress in my feet

- I now relax and let go of any tension and stress in my calves

- I now relax and let go of any tension and stress in my thighs and hips

- I now relax and let go of any tension and stress in my stomach

- I now relax and let go of any tension and stress in my back

- I now relax and let go of any tension and stress in my chest

- I now relax and let go of any tension and stress in my shoulders

- I now relax and let go of any tension and stress in my arms and hands

- I now relax and let go of any tension and stress in my neck

- I now relax and let go of any tension and stress in my face and head

- My whole body is now calm and relaxed

"The greatest healing therapy is friendship and love."

- Hubert Humphrey

"A strong positive mental attitude will create more miracles than any wonder drug."

-Patricia Neal

Chapter Six

Guidelines

This chapter presents the basic guidelines for doing a Cancer Guided Imagery session. These guidelines are not cast in stone, but have been proven to be the most effective. If you feel the need to change or adjust any guidelines, feel free to do so. The bottom line is to do what works and feels comfortable for you. The key to successful Cancer Guided Imagery sessions is to be flexible and have an open mind.

Guidelines

➤ The number one guideline for all Cancer Guided Imagery is ensuring that all suggestions are focused on your cancer treatment and recovery.

➤ At the beginning of each Cancer Guided Imagery session, assume an attitude of acceptance and openness towards it. Intend to put forth the best effort possible;

nothing more, and nothing less. It's that simple. This might seem difficult to do at first. If you are having a hard time, follow the AA (Alcoholics Anonymous) saying, "fake it 'til you make it." Just go through the process with the intent of openness and acceptance that was mentioned before. Soon the acceptance and openness will become automatic with each session.

➢ Imagery Content does not have to be physiologically correct for it to produce results. This means that precise knowledge of how the immune system functions or any other part of the body is not required. It is really not necessary for you to be an expert on the human body and cancer. But, knowledge and/or an overview of your type of cancer, treatment and recovery is recommended. This knowledge will help enhance Cancer Guided Imagery sessions.

➢ Imagery Content should always be personalized. The most effective images created are those that have specific and personal meaning to the individual.

➢ Always personalize circumstances, events, places, and people when doing Cancer Guided Imagery. The Imagery Content used during Cancer Guided Imagery should truly be your own.

➢ Imagery Content should always be aligned with your personal values and beliefs. Never use Imagery Content that doesn't feel right. Learn to trust your feelings and intuition. If the Imagery Content feels right, do not worry, use it! It can always be changed in later sessions.

➢ You can share your Cancer Guided Imagery Content with others, if you like. Just remember, universal meanings from books and/or other people's interpretations of your Imagery Content can be very subjective. Although this feedback may be useful for guidance and suggestions, stay with your own interpretations.

Additional Guidelines

➢ Make sure that all Cancer Guided Imagery suggestions and Imagery Content are always positive and reflect your well-being.

➢ Try to do a Cancer Guided Imagery session at least every other day for the first 60 days. This will help develop your skill with Cancer Guided Imagery. It also allows your body to receive many positive messages over the first 60 days. If a day or two is missed, do not worry; just continue the next session when the time is available. You can do as many sessions as you desire or have the time for. After the first 60 days, sessions can be performed on your own schedule or as needed.

➢ Most people find at first it is easier to do Cancer Guided Imagery in the morning or at night before going to bed. With practice you will be able to do it whenever and wherever there is an opportunity.

➤ In the beginning sessions of Cancer Guided Imagery, everyone is at different levels of ability. Do not worry about your level when you start, after several weeks of doing sessions, your level of ability will greatly increase.

➤ After a Cancer Guided Imagery session if you have the time, you can sit quietly and contemplate or reflect upon it. This is not required, but some people find this helpful for future sessions.

➤ One can write notes, or make drawings of what transpired during the session. This information can be used to make adjustments to the Imagery Content for the next session and/or to keep a record of your progress.

"Human beings, by changing the inner attitudes of their minds, can change the outer aspects of their lives."

-William James

"Change your thoughts and you change your world."

-Norman Vincent Peale

Chapter Seven

Step-by-Step Directions

This chapter provides directions for doing a Cancer Guided Imagery session. Everyone and their circumstances are different. With that in mind, one may have to modify and/or adjust the directions. Read the directions a minimum of four times before the first session. Write down a list of the steps or notes to help during early sessions until the process is memorized.

Step-by Step

➤ Set aside enough time when doing a Cancer Guided Imagery session so you are not rushed. When you first start you will need to allocate additional time for a session. After you become experienced with the process, you will be able to adjust the time accordingly.

➤ Cancer Guided Imagery works best in a relaxed, quiet setting. Find a room or an area with soft lighting and no disturbances. Make sure there is a comfortable place to sit or lie down. Loosen clothing and remove shoes. You can lie down, but sitting up, if possible, is recommended.

➤ Soothing, calm background music can also be incorporated, but it isn't necessary. Do make sure that any music played is not loud or distracting. Music, when properly chosen, will increase the effects of your session. You will intuitively know what music is right. Some people prefer no music at all and that is OK.

➤ Have an open mind and do not get up tight about "doing it right." Remember to just do the best you can each session.

➤ It is suggested you do one Cancer Guided Imagery session once every other day for the first 60 days. This provides enough practice and experience with the process to develop a solid mind and body connection.

➤ Cancer Guided Imagery sessions can be done as many as three times a day or more, depending on your needs, time, and circumstances.

➤ If a session is missed for any reason, that's OK! Just do the next session as soon as possible. The every other day for 60 consecutive days guideline is not set in stone; it's just an optimum direction. Some people, due to their circumstances, might only be able to do it every third day. After the 60 days you can set up a schedule that works best for you.

➤ Prior to a session, write down or make copies from the book of the suggestions and Imagery Content as reminders to use throughout the session. This is easier than trying to remember them, and they will always be in the correct sequence. If the Imagery Content is being acquired unconsciously during the session, then only the suggestions will be written down.

➤ Another option is to have a relative or friend present during one's sessions. They can serve as a guide, or helper. They can read the suggestions and the Imagery Content to you. Some people prefer to do all of their sessions this way, or just a few. You might find it helpful to record the suggestions and Imagery Content, instead of writing it down or having it read to you. When recording Imagery Content and suggestions, be sure to include a ten second pause between each one. This way, after each suggestion and Imagery Content, the recorder can be paused, and the next suggestion and Imagery Content is queued up.

➤ On occasion, you may fall asleep during a session. If that happens, when you awaken, simply resume where you left off. Or just continue the session at another time.

➢ In the beginning, it is normal to "space out" or have a wandering mind during a Cancer Guided Imagery session. When this happens, just gently re –focus your thoughts back to the session, and continue on. With practice and experience, this will happen less and less.

➢ It's always good to have tissues close by during sessions. On occasion Cancer Guided Imagery will sometimes elicit emotions. You might tear up and/ or get a runny nose. This is a positive sign, which demonstrates that the Imagery Content is being communicated to the body. If this does happen, do not worry about these physical responses; they are normal, just continue on. If you feel the need to stop for the day, do it–not a problem. Perform the next Cancer Guided Imagery session as scheduled.

➢ You can stop a Cancer Guided Imagery session anytime, for any reason and there is no harm. Just start where you left off or at the beginning in the next session.

➢ The eyes may be open or closed during a Cancer Guided Imagery session. Individuals who do not visualize well, often keep their eyes open and look at a peaceful image. If the eyes remain open, you can gaze at an appealing painting, a photo of a nature scene, a candle, or just focus on a place in the room where the eyes can rest. If closing the eyes is more comfortable, do so. There is not a right or a wrong way regarding the eyes; it is what works best for you. Try both ways or even do a combination of both. If the eyes are closed and the suggestions and Imagery Content are written down or taped, of course open them to read or use the tape recorder.

➤ At first, completing a suggestion and its Imagery Content may take a while. Do not worry; the time will vary with early sessions. Once you become experienced at doing Cancer Guided Imagery, each suggestion and its Imagery Content ideally should not take longer than two to three minutes to complete. This is plenty of time for the mind to process the Imagery Content and communicate it to the body. Once you are experienced in the process, ten suggestions during one Cancer Guided Imagery session should take about 30 minutes to finish. This does not include doing the Relaxation Technique at the beginning. Two to three minutes might not seem like enough time for a suggestion, and it might not be at first, but with practice, it is generally plenty of time. You eventually develop awareness for how long a session takes to complete.

➤ Generate as much positive enthusiasm as you can during a session. Depending on your mood and circumstances your intensity level might vary from session to session. This is normal, do not worry if this happens. As I said many times before, just do the best you can during each session.

➤ Always state a suggestion out loud or silently before acquiring the Imagery Content for it.

➤ Allow at least a 30 second pause between each suggestion to clear the mind of the previous Imagery Content before moving to the next suggestion. When a suggestion is completed, say silently or out loud: "clear the mind" or "clear," then wait the 30 seconds.

Cancer Guided Imagery Suggestions

Cancer Guided Imagery suggestions that ask you to be "prepared," should always include two parts to the Imagery Content. For example, "I imagine myself *prepared* emotionally for a successful treatment." I will explain the two parts of this suggestion.

The first part of the Imagery Content for this suggestion has to include what you personally need to do to prepare for a successful treatment. There is flexibility and personalization with this Imagery Content because everyone will require different ways to prepare emotionally for their treatment.

The second part of the Imagery Content has to include a successful completion of the first part. In other words imagine what needs to be done, then imagine doing it successfully. By imagining both parts of the Imagery Content, you are then *prepared* for a successful treatment through Cancer Guided Imagery. Once again, it is very important with Imagery Suggestions that ask you to be "prepared," to have two parts of Imagery Content.

There are Cancer Guided Imagery suggestions that can be done with only one segment of the Imagery Content. For example, "I imagine myself physically strong." One could simply acquire Imagery Content based on his or her perception of being physically strong. This Imagery Content could be something like walking briskly in a park, hiking, or doing any activity that requires physical strength. Or it could be just imagery of the person looking and being physically strong, without doing an activity.

This type of suggestion could also be done in two segments. The first part would be images of looking very physically strong; the second part would be imagery doing an activity that requires physical strength.

Ultimately you have to decide if a suggestion needs two parts for the Imagery Content. Usually this will be determined by the way the suggestion is phrased. All suggestions should be structured to give flexibility in acquiring Imagery Content.

Example of a Suggestion

You can use one or up to ten suggestions during a Cancer Guided Imagery session. Let's follow one suggestion, "I imagine myself peaceful and calm during my Radiation treatment," through the entire process.

First, it's decided to acquire the Imagery Content for the suggestion consciously as described in a previous chapter. Hence, you are prepared with the Imagery Content for this suggestion before the session begins. The suggestion is written down, with a few notes on the Imagery Content to be used.

A quiet environment with or without music in the background is needed. The eyes can be opened or closed. If they are open, you are gazing at a picture of a calm nature scene. The suggestions and notes for the Imagery Content are close by so you can read them. Begin with the Relaxation Technique, and then proceed to the Cancer Guided Imagery suggestions. Read the first suggestion, "I imagine myself peaceful and calm during my Radiation treatment," out loud or silently. Then refer to the notes for the Imagery Content and then proceed with the imagery for it.

Let's say the Imagery Content you have for this suggestion is just one segment. It is of you in a clean orderly room, surrounded by professional medical people, state of the art medical equipment and you are receiving a Radiation treatment. While receiving the treatment you are peaceful and calm.

Your Imagery Content can have as many details as you are able to imagine. The most essential aspect of this Imagery Content is that it reflects you being peaceful and calm during the Radiation treatment.

Maybe when you are doing the imagery you can imagine the environment and the people during your treatment clearly, but you can imagine yourself only slightly calm and peaceful. That is OK, just do the best you can for the two to three minutes and then move to the next suggestion. Please do not worry or dwell upon this. Each session builds on the previous session and has an accumulative effect, so you will improve.

Ideally you complete the Imagery Content for this suggestion in two to three minutes. You then state, "clear," silently or out loud and wait for about 30 seconds before continuing to the next suggestion, starting the same process over again.

"Imagination is more important than knowledge."

-Albert Einstein

Chapter Eight

Cancer Guided Imagery Sessions

The following chapters contain Cancer Guided Imagery sessions on Chemotherapy, Radiation, Surgery, Cancer Recovery and Dissolving and Destroying Cancer Cells. These Cancer Guided Imagery sessions, which include corresponding suggestions, will deliver multiple layers of helpful messages to the body that build on one another and lay a strong, deeply ingrained foundation for successful Cancer Treatment and Recovery.

Each session has ten suggestions that are organized and listed in a logical sequence. However, if you desire, feel free to change the sequence of a few suggestions, or even some of the suggestions themselves. There is also an affirmation for each suggestion that can be used as an alternative for the two ways described and explained in a previous chapter.

All the suggestions can be completed in one session, or do as many as time and circumstances permit. If any suggestions cannot be completed in a session, just begin where you left off in the next session.

The Cancer Guided Imagery sessions in the following chapters are just guides. But, I highly recommend that they be used for your first sessions. After the first sessions they can continue to be used. Or you can modify them depending on the needs and circumstances of your cancer treatment and recovery. You can develop new Cancer Guided Imagery suggestions for your sessions. Just remember to list the suggestions in a logical sequence for treatment and/or recovery during your session. Use the same method for acquiring Imagery Content for these new suggestions.

As a final reminder, remember to always perform the Relaxation Technique before each Cancer Guided Imagery session.

"Everything you can imagine is real."

-Pablo Picasso

"The greatest discovery of my generation is that a human being can alter his life by altering his attitudes of mind."

-William James

Chapter Nine

Cancer Surgery

Relaxation

Take five to ten deep breaths. When you exhale on each breath, say out loud or think the word "relax."

After the five to ten breaths, just breathe at a normal pace and stop thinking or saying the word relax when you exhale.

State each body part direction out loud or silently before you relax it.

• I now relax and let go of any tension and stress in my feet

• I now relax and let go of any tension and stress in my calves

- I now relax and let go of any tension and stress in my thighs and hips

- I now relax and let go of any tension and stress in my stomach

- I now relax and let go of any tension and stress in my back

- I now relax and let go of any tension and stress in my chest

- I now relax and let go of any tension and stress in my shoulders

- I now relax and let go of any tension and stress in my arms and hands

- I now relax and let go of any tension and stress in my neck

- I now relax and let go of any tension and stress in my face and head

- My whole body is now calm and relaxed

Cancer Guided Imagery

1. Suggestion – I imagine myself prepared emotionally for my surgery

Affirmation – I am prepared emotionally for my surgery

2. Suggestion – I imagine myself prepared mentally for my surgery

Affirmation – I am prepared mentally for my surgery

3. Suggestion – I imagine myself prepared physically for my surgery

Affirmation – I am prepared physically for my surgery

4. Suggestion – I imagine myself peaceful and calm before my surgery

Affirmation – I am peaceful and calm before my surgery

5. Suggestion – I imagine my vital body signs being stable during my surgery

Affirmation – My vital body signs are stable during my surgery

6. Suggestion – I imagine my doctor performing successful surgery

Affirmation – My doctor will perform successful surgery

7. Suggestion – I imagine myself with minimal discomfort after my surgery

Affirmation – I have minimal discomfort after my surgery

8. Suggestion – I imagine my surgery completely successful

Affirmation – My surgery is completely successful

9. Suggestion – I imagine all my incisions healed completely

Affirmation – All my incisions are healed completely

10. Suggestion – I imagine my body and mind completely healed

Affirmation – My body and mind are completely healed

Notes, New Suggestions and Affirmations

"Imagination is the beginning of creation. You imagine what you desire, you will what you imagine and at last you create what you will."

-George Bernard Shaw

Chapter Ten

Destroying & Dissolving Cancer Cells

Relaxation

Take five to ten deep breaths. When you exhale on each breath, say out loud or think the word "relax."

After the five to ten breaths, just breathe at a normal pace and stop thinking or saying the word relax when you exhale.

State each body part direction out loud or silently before you relax it.

- I now relax and let go of any tension and stress in my feet

- I now relax and let go of any tension and stress in my calves

- I now relax and let go of any tension and stress in my thighs and hips

- I now relax and let go of any tension and stress in my stomach

- I now relax and let go of any tension and stress in my back

- I now relax and let go of any tension and stress in my chest

- I now relax and let go of any tension and stress in my shoulders

- I now relax and let go of any tension and stress in my arms and hands

- I now relax and let go of any tension and stress in my neck

- I now relax and let go of any tension and stress in my face and head

- My whole body is now calm and relaxed

Cancer Guided Imagery

1. Suggestion – I imagine my immune system strong and powerful throughout my body

Affirmation – My immune system is strong and powerful throughout my body

2. Suggestion – I imagine what my cancer cells look like

Affirmation – I know what my cancer cells look like

3. Suggestion – I imagine my cancer cells being weak and confused

Affirmation – My cancer cells are weak and confused

4. Suggestion – I imagine what my white blood cells look like

Affirmation – I know what my white blood cells look like

5. Suggestion – I imagine my white blood cells being very powerful and strong, surging throughout my body

Affirmation – My white blood cells are powerful and strong, surging throughout my body

6. Suggestion – I imagine my immune system releasing a large army of white blood cells throughout my body

Affirmation – I have released a large army of white blood cells throughout my body

7. Suggestion – I imagine this large army finding cancer cells and destroying and dissolving them

Affirmation – This large army finds cancer cells and destroys and dissolves them

8. Suggestion – I imagine the dissolved and destroyed cancer cells being flushed from my body

Affirmation – My dissolved and destroyed cancer cells are being flushed from my body

9. Suggestion – I imagine my healthy cells repairing any damage throughout my body

Affirmation – My healthy cells have repaired any damage throughout my body

10. Suggestion – I imagine my body and mind completely healed

Affirmation – My body and mind are completely healed

Notes, New Suggestions and Affirmations

"The universe is change; our life is what our thoughts make it."

-Marcus Aurelius Antoninus

Chapter Eleven

Chemotherapy

Relaxation

Take five to ten deep breaths. When you exhale on each breath, say out loud or think the word "relax."

After the five to ten breaths, just breathe at a normal pace and stop thinking or saying the word relax when you exhale.

State each body part direction out loud or silently before you relax it.

• I now relax and let go of any tension and stress in my feet

• I now relax and let go of any tension and stress in my calves

- I now relax and let go of any tension and stress in my thighs and hips

- I now relax and let go of any tension and stress in my stomach

- I now relax and let go of any tension and stress in my back

- I now relax and let go of any tension and stress in my chest

- I now relax and let go of any tension and stress in my shoulders

- I now relax and let go of any tension and stress in my arms and hands

- I now relax and let go of any tension and stress in my neck

- I now relax and let go of any tension and stress in my face and head

- My whole body is now calm and relaxed

Cancer Guided Imagery

1. Suggestion – I imagine myself prepared emotionally for my Chemotherapy

Affirmation – I am prepared emotionally for my Chemotherapy

2. Suggestion – I imagine myself prepared mentally for my Chemotherapy

Affirmation – I am prepared mentally for my Chemotherapy

3. Suggestion – I imagine myself prepared physically for my Chemotherapy

Affirmation – I am prepared physically for my Chemotherapy

4. Suggestion – I imagine myself peaceful and calm during my Chemotherapy

Affirmation – I am peaceful and calm during my Chemotherapy

5. Suggestion – I imagine my cancer cells being dissolved and destroyed during my Chemotherapy.

Affirmation – My cancer cells are dissolved and destroyed during my Chemotherapy

6. Suggestion – I imagine my remaining cells healthy throughout my body

Affirmation – My remaining cells are healthy throughout my body

7. Suggestion – I imagine myself with minimal discomfort after my Chemotherapy

Affirmation – I have minimal discomfort after my Chemotherapy

8. Suggestion – I imagine myself with energy after my Chemotherapy

Affirmation – I have energy after my chemotherapy

9. Suggestion – I imagine my Chemotherapy is successful

Affirmation – My Chemotherapy is successful

10. Suggestion – I imagine my body and mind completely healed

Affirmation – My body and mind are completely healed

Notes, New Suggestions and Affirmations

"There is only one admirable form of the imagination: the imagination that is so intense that it creates a new reality, that it makes things happen."

-Sean O'Faolain

Chapter Twelve

Radiation

Relaxation

Take five to ten deep breaths. When you exhale on each breath, say out loud or think the word "relax."

After the five to ten breaths, just breathe at a normal pace and stop thinking or saying the word relax when you exhale.

State each body part direction out loud or silently before you relax it.

- I now relax and let go of any tension and stress in my feet

- I now relax and let go of any tension and stress in my calves

- I now relax and let go of any tension and stress in my thighs and hips

- I now relax and let go of any tension and stress in my stomach

- I now relax and let go of any tension and stress in my back

- I now relax and let go of any tension and stress in my chest

- I now relax and let go of any tension and stress in my shoulders

- I now relax and let go of any tension and stress in my arms and hands

- I now relax and let go of any tension and stress in my neck

- I now relax and let go of any tension and stress in my face and head

- My whole body is now calm and relaxed

Cancer Guided Imagery

1. Suggestion – I imagine myself prepared emotionally for my Radiation treatment

Affirmation – I am prepared emotionally for my Radiation treatment

2. Suggestion – I imagine myself prepared mentally for my Radiation treatment

Affirmation – I am prepared mentally for my Radiation treatment

3. Suggestion – I imagine myself prepared physically for my Radiation treatment

Affirmation – I am prepared physically for my Radiation treatment

4. Suggestion – I imagine myself peaceful and calm during my Radiation treatment

Affirmation – I am peaceful and calm during my radiation treatment

5. Suggestion – I imagine my cancer cells burned and dissolved during my radiation treatment

Affirmation – My cancer cells are burned and dissolved during my radiation treatment

6. Suggestion – I imagine my remaining cells healthy throughout my body

Affirmation – My remaining cells are healthy throughout my body

7. Suggestion – I imagine myself with minimal discomfort after my Radiation treatment

Affirmation – I have minimal discomfort after my Radiation treatment

8. Suggestion – I imagine myself with energy after my Radiation treatment

Affirmation – I have energy after my Radiation treatment

9. Suggestion – I imagine my Radiation treatment successful

Affirmation – My Radiation treatment is successful

10. Suggestion – I imagine my body and mind completely healed

Affirmation – My body and mind are completely healed

Notes, New Suggestions and Affirmations

"Love cures people — both the ones who give it and the ones who receive it."

-Dr. Karl Menninger

Chapter Thirteen

Cancer Recovery

Relaxation

Take five to ten deep breaths. When you exhale on each breath, say out loud or think the word "relax."

After the five to ten breaths, just breathe at a normal pace and stop thinking or saying the word relax when you exhale.

State each body part direction out loud or silently before you relax it.

• I now relax and let go of any tension and stress in my feet

• I now relax and let go of any tension and stress in my calves

- I now relax and let go of any tension and stress in my thighs and hips

- I now relax and let go of any tension and stress in my stomach

- I now relax and let go of any tension and stress in my back

- I now relax and let go of any tension and stress in my chest

- I now relax and let go of any tension and stress in my shoulders

- I now relax and let go of any tension and stress in my arms and hands

- I now relax and let go of any tension and stress in my neck

- I now relax and let go of any tension and stress in my face and head

- My whole body is now calm and relaxed

Cancer Guided Imagery

1. Suggestion – I imagine all my cancer treatments successful

Affirmation – All my cancer treatments are successful

2. Suggestion – I imagine myself mentally stronger each day

Affirmation – I am mentally stronger each day

3. Suggestion – I imagine myself emotionally stronger each day

Affirmation – I am emotionally stronger each day

4. Suggestion – I imagine myself physically stronger each day

Affirmation – I am physically stronger each day

5. Suggestion – I imagine what I must do to maintain my health

Affirmation – I am doing what I must do to maintain my health

6. Suggestion – I imagine myself returning to my daily activities

Affirmation – I am returning to my daily activities

7. Suggestion – I imagine myself having fun with family and friends

Affirmation – I am having fun with family and friends

8. Suggestion – I imagine myself achieving my goals in life

Affirmation – I am achieving my goals in life

9. Suggestion – I imagine my immune system healthy throughout my body

Affirmation – My immune system is healthy throughout my body

10. Suggestion – I imagine my body and mind completely healed

Affirmation – My body and mind are completely healed

Notes, New Suggestions and Affirmations

Chapter 13 Cancer Recovery

INDEX

SELECTED BIBLIOGRAPHY

Rossman, M.L. *Guided Imagery for Self-Healing.* H J Kramer and New World Library, 2000. *(Footnote 1)*

Simonton, Carl O. MD, Simonton, S., Creighton, J.L. *Getting Well Again.* Bantam Books, 1978. ISBN: 0553280333 *(Footnote 7)*

McNaughten, H. *Emile Coue: The Man and His Work.* ISBN:1858101042 *(Footnote 11)*

Benson, H. MD. *The Relaxation Response.* 1975. ISBN: 0380815958 *(Footnote 12)*

Weinstein, L. *Creative Imagery in Nursing.* Delmar Publishers, 1996. ISBN: 082736394

Shone, R. *Creative Visualization: Using Imagery and Imagination for Self-Transformation.* Destiny Books, 1998. ISBN : 089281707.

Holden, M. *Healing Images for Children: Teaching Relaxation and Guided Imagery to Children Facing Cancer and Other Serious Illnesses.* Inner Coaching, 2001. ISBN: 0963602721.

Brigham, DD. *Imagery for Getting Well: Clinical Applications of behavioral Medicine.* Norton & Co., 1996. ISBN: 0393702251.

Naparstek, B. *Staying Well With Guided Imagery.* Warner Books, 1995. ISBN: 0446671347.

Achterberg, J. Ph.D., L. *Rituals of Healing: Using Imagery for Health and Wellness.* Bantam Books, 1994. ISBN: 0553373471

Fezler, W. Ph.D.*Creative Imagery: How to Visualize in All Five Senses.* Fireside Books, 1989. ISBN: 0671682385

Epstein, G.MD.*Healing Visualizations: Creating Health Through Imagery.* Bantam Books, 1989. ISBN: 0553346237.

King, S. *Imagineering for Health.* Quest Books. ISBN 0835605469

CANCER HELP & SUPPORT GROUPS

- Coalition of National Cancer Cooperative Groups, Inc.
Provides cancer clinical trials and research.
www.Cancertrialshelp.org
1818 Market Street #1100
Philadelphia, PA 19103
Phone: 1-877-520-4457
Fax: 215-789-3655

-NABCO National Alliance of Breast Cancer Organizations
www.nabco.org/index.php/20
NABCO Regional Support Group Database from across the country.
9 East 37th Street, 10th Floor
New York, NY 10016
Phone: 212-889-0606 / 888-80-NABCO
Fax: 212-689-1213

-National Cancer Institute
Patient Education Branch Cancer Support Groups:
Questions and Answers
www.cancer.gov
6116 Executive Blvd. Suite 202
Bethesda, MD 20892-8334
Phone: 301-451-4065 / toll free 1-800-4-CANCER

-American Cancer Society
www.cancer.org
1-800-ACS-2345

-The National Coalition of Cancer Survivorship-NCCS
Survivor-led advocacy organization working exclusively on behalf of
people with all types of cancer and their families, is dedicated to assuring
quality cancer care for all Americans.
www.canceradvocacy.org
877-NCCS-YES (622-7937)
1010 Wayne Avenue Suite 770
Silver Spring, MD 20910
Phone: 301-650-9127
Fax: 301-565-9670

-Kids Konnected
Support for kids with parent(s) with cancer
www.kidskonnected.org
27071 Cabot Road Suite 102
Laguna Hills, CA 92653
Phone: 949-582-5443

-Y-ME National Breast Cancer Organization
212 W. Van Buren Suite 500
Chicago, IL 60607
Phone: 312-986-8338

-Cancer News
www.cancernews.com
Cancer News on the net is dedicated to brining patients and their families
the latest news and information on cancer diagnosis, treatment and
prevention. This service is offered for free.

-International Union Against Cancer
International groups for cancer info and support
www.uicc.org

-Association of American Cancer Institutes
www.aaci-cancer.org
200 Lothrop Street
Iroquois Building Suite 305
Pittsburgh, PA 15213
Phone: 412-647-2076
Fax: 412-647-3659

-Cancer Centers and Institutes
Guide to Internet Resources for Cancer
www.cancerindex.org

-A.P. John Institute for Cancer Research
Cancer Treatment, Prevention and Research
www.apjohncancerinstitute.org
67 Arch Street
Greenwich Ct. 06830
Phone: 203-661-2571
Fax: 203-629-0966

-Tulane Cancer Center
Cancer treatment and research
www.canceriscurable.com
Tulane Cancer Center, Box SL-68
1430 Tulane Avenue
New Orleans, Louisiana 70112-2699
Phone: 504-585-6060
Fax: 504-585-6077

-Cancer Research Institute
Exploring the body's immune system as a way to prevent, control, and
cure cancer
www.cancerresearch.org
681 Fifth Avenue
New York, NY 10022
Phone: 1-800-99CANCER or
        1-800-992-2623

-What you need to know about cancer
www.cancer.about.com/cs/supportgroups/info

**-ALCASE Alliance for Lung Cancer Advocacy, Support, and
Education**
www.alcase.org/support/suprtgrps.html
ALCASE is the only not-for-profit organization dedicated solely to
helping those living with lung cancer to improve the quality of their lives
through support and education.
Phone: 360-696-2436
Fax: 360-735-1305
Lung Cancer Hotline: 1-800-298-2436
Email: info @alcase.org

-Support Group Links
http://www.cancerindex.org/clinks6a.htm

-Support and Resources Cancer.gov
http://www.nci.nih.gov/cancer_information/support/
1-800-4-cancer
Information about cancer support organizations, finances, insurance,
hospice care and home care.

-The Cancer Patients Aid Association (CPAA) information for aid for cancer patients.
http://216.122.199.245/SupportGroup/cancer/index.asp

-Shared Experience Cancer Support Site
www.sharedexperience.org
Cancer patients share stories and case histories bulletin board.

-Breast Cancer Support Groups
www.womenshealth.org/a/breastcancersupportgroups.htm

-Virtual Wellness Community on line support groups
www.thewellnesscommunity.org/virtual_WC/support.htm
National Offices:
919 18th Street NW Suite 54
Washington, DC 20006
Toll Free: 1-888-793-WELL
Email: help@thewellnesscommunity.org

-Breast Support Groups Search Engine for USA
www.hersource.com/breast/06/6b/supportgroup.cfm
A safe place to meet people to talk about your experience dealing with breast cancer and search for local support groups.
Email: support.breastcancer@nexcura.com

-Share self-help for women with breast cancer or ovarian cancer
www.sharecancersupport.org/pages/02Programs/programs07_01.html
Phone: 212-719-0364
1-866-891-2392

-US TOO! International
Prostate Cancer Education and Support Group Chapters
www.ustoo.com/chapters.html
1-800-80-US TOO (800-808-7866)
Chicago area: 630-795-1002 9am-4: 30pm CT

RESEARCH AND REFERENCE

FOOTNOTES

2 - Dr. Alan Watkins states that every idea, thought and belief has a neurochemical consequence, which is what makes imagery such a significant mind-body bridge. He writes that the flow of neuropeptides from the CNS, which enhances or inhibits one's immunology through two major neuro immuno modulatory pathways; neuroendocrine and autonomic, are critically important in maintaining health and fighting disease [Watkins A 1997 Mind-body medicine. Churchill Livingstone, NY].

3 - D. L. Tusek and R. E. Cwynar of Ohio acknowledged that patients often describe the experience in a hospital as overwhelming, evoking fear, anger, helplessness, and isolation. Tusek and Cwynar view guided imagery as one of the most well-studied complementary therapies being used that can improve the patient experience and outcome by providing a significant source of strength, support, and courage as they prepare for a procedure or manage the stresses of a hospital stay [AACN Clin Issues 2000 Feb; 11(1): 68-76].

4 - V. W. Donaldson in NC at the Center for Stress Management examined the effects of mental imagery on the immune system response, and specifically, on depressed white blood cell (WBC) counts. Results indicated significant increases in WBC count for all patients over a 90-day period, even when possessing disease and illnesses that would have predicted a decrease in WBC count [Appl Psychophysiol Biofeedback 2000 Jun; 25(2): 117-28].

5 - L. M. Troesch et al. of the Arthur G. James Cancer Hospital and Research Institute at Ohio State University in Columbus found that those patients using a chemotherapy-specific guided-imagery audiotape expressed a significantly more positive experience with chemotherapy, finding guided imagery to be an effective intervention to promote patient involvement in self-care practices and to increase patient coping abilities during symptom occurrence [Oncol Nurs Forum 1993 Sep; 20(8): 1179-85].

6 - D. S. Burns at the Group/Walther Cancer Institute found that individuals who participated in guided imagery sessions scored better on both mood scores and quality of life scores than those who did not. Interestingly, these scores continued to improve in the experimental group, even after sessions were complete, indicating that guided imagery is effective in improving mood and quality of life in cancer patients [J. Music Ther. 2001 spring; 38(1) :51-65].

8 - Gaston-Johansson et al. of Johns Hopkins University School of Nursing in Baltimore, Maryland showed significant benefits from the use of information, cognitive restructuring, and relaxation with guided imagery in those patients with breast cancer who underwent autologous bone marrow/peripheral blood stem cell transplantation. This strategy was found to be effective in significantly reducing anxiety, nausea, and nausea combined with fatigue 7 days after surgery when the side effects of treatment are usually the most severe [Cancer Nurs 2000 Aug; 23(4):277-85].

9 - Researchers at Ohio State University in Columbus, Ohio found that people with cancer who used imagery while receiving chemotherapy felt more relaxed, better prepared for their treatment and more positive about care than those who didn't use the technique. They also found it can help chemotherapy patients cope with one of the most severe side effects of their treatment.

10 - Howard Hall, measuring the effects of healthy people imagining their White blood cells as strong as powerful sharks, found a number of subjects could demonstrate an increase in the number of lymphocytes as well as an increased responsiveness of the immune system after the session as compared to before [Hall H R 1983 Hypnosis and the immune system. American Journal of Clinical Hypnosis, 25:92-103].

13 - C. H. McKinney et al. from the University of Miami found that 13 weeks of guided imagery and music showed significant decreases in cortisol level (the "stress hormone" strongly correlated with mood disturbances, as well as demonstrating a significant reduction in depression, fatigue, and total mood disturbance.) The study also [Health Psychol 1997 Jul; 16(4): 390-400].

Fear

L. Baider, et al. examined the long-term effects of relaxation and guided imagery on patients recently diagnosed with cancer at Hadassah University Hospital. Results showed a decrease in psychological distress and an increase in the patient's sense of internal control [Gen Hosp Psychiatry 2001 Sep-Oct; 23(5): 272-7].

A study by J. A. Royle, et al. of Ontario, found that guided imagery was the intervention best used by nurses to decrease patient anxiety [Can Oncol Nurs J 1996 Feb; 6(1): 20-5].

Depression

Fawzy et al. found that information on the cancer and training in stress management and coping skills, showed participants exhibiting less fatigue, depression, mood disturbances, as well as increased vigor [Fawzy F I, Kemeny M E, Fawzy N W et al. 1990 A structured psychiatric intervention for cancer patients: II. Changes over time in immunological measures. Archive of General Psychiatry 47:729-35].

B. L. Rees reported that patients receiving 4 weeks of relaxation and guided imagery scored significantly lower on trait anxiety, state anxiety, and depression, while scoring significantly higher on measurements of self-esteem [J. of Holistic Nursing. 13(3): 255-267. Sept. 1995].

C.L. Norred at the University of Colorado Health Sciences Center Department of Anesthesiology in Denver found that guided imagery may be an integrative therapy that can minimize preoperative anxiety [AORN J 2000 Nov; 72(5): 838-40, 842-3].

S.A. Lambert found that guided imagery and relaxation therapy significantly lowered postoperative pain ratings and shortened the hospital stays, as well as decreased the postoperative anxiety [J Dev Behav Pediatr 1996 Oct; 17(5): 307-10].

Anxiety-Quality of Life

C. H. McKinney et al. from the University of Miami found that 13 weeks of guided imagery and music showed significant decreases in cortisol level (the "stress hormone" strongly correlated with mood disturbances, as well as demonstrating a significant reduction in depression, fatigue, and total mood disturbance. The study also [Health Psychol 1997 Jul; 16(4): 390-400].

B. L. Rees reported that patients receiving 4 weeks of relaxation and guided imagery scored significantly lower on trait anxiety, state anxiety, and depression, while scoring significantly higher on measurements of self-esteem [J. of Holistic Nursing. 13(3): 255-267. Sept. 1995].

L. G. Walker et al. of the University of Aberdeen Medical School found that cancer patients receiving standard care plus relaxation training and imagery were more relaxed and easy going during the study, experiencing a higher quality of life overall during primary chemotherapy [Br J Cancer 1999 Apr; 80(1-2): 262-8].

A study by J. A. Royle, et al. of Ontario, found that guided imagery was the best intervention used by nurses to decrease patient anxiety [Can Oncol Nurs J 1996 Feb; 6(1): 20-5].

Side Effects-Pain

K.L. Syrjala et al. of the Fred Hutchinson Cancer Research Center in Seattle, WA concluded in their study that stand-alone relaxation and imagery training reduces cancer treatment-related pain [Pain 1995 Nov; 63(2): 189-98].

R.Sloman from the University of Sydney in Australia observed that progressive muscle relaxation combined with guided imagery has the potential to promote relief of cancer pain. The techniques appear to produce a relaxation response that may break the pain-muscle-tension-anxiety cycle and facilitate pain relief through a calming effect. This technique seems to provide a self-care strategy that, to a limited extent, shifts the locus of control from clinician to patient [Nurs Clin North Am 1995 Dec; 30(4): 697-709].

R. J. Moore and D. Spiegel from the Anderson Cancer Center in Houston, TX observed a desire for and a benefit from patients being able to attach meaning to the disease and its treatment. They felt that this is why many are drawn to guided imagery as a tool in the management of cancer-related anxiety and pain by using it to reconnect to the self, to make sense of their experiences with breast cancer, and for managing cancer pain in a manner that increases one's sense of control, thereby alleviating the suffering of the survivor [1096-2190 2000 Mar 21; 2(2): 115-126].

D.L. Tusek, R. Cwynar, and D.M. Cosgrove studied the effect of listening to taped guided imagery for patients undergoing cardiovascular surgeries and concluded that guided imagery can decrease length of stay, pain, and anxiety [J of Cardiovascular Management. 22-28. March-April 1999].

C Renzi et al. found that listening to guided imagery tapes before, during, and after surgery showed results in which there was a trend for reduction in pain following surgery and a significant improvement in the quality of sleep [Int J Colorectal Dis 2000 Nov; 15(5-6): 313-6].

Omlor et al. found that preoperative relaxation techniques significantly reduced the number of postoperative hematomas as well as the amount of pain medication being required after surgery [Zentralbl Chir 2000; 125(4): 380-5; discussion 385-6].

Journal of Consulting and Clinical Psychology: 1991 Aug; 59(4): 518-25 concluded that relaxation therapy is effective in reducing adverse consequences of chemotherapy, for a study involving 81 cancer patients showed relaxation therapy to decrease nausea and anxiety during chemotherapy.

K. L. Kaufman et al. at Ohio State University tried a self-hypnotic, cue-controlled relaxation, and guided imagery intervention that showed a marked and clinically significant reduction in nausea and vomiting as well as a concurrent increase in sleep duration [J Adolesc Health Care 1989 Jul; 10(4): 323-7].

Immune Response

K. Glaser and R. Glaser, studying a group of elderly people, found that over a month of relaxation training three times per week significantly increased their natural killer lymphocytes and T cell activity [Cousins N 1989 Head first. Dutton, NY].

J. Pennebaker found that "confessional writing," of the type that occurs when journaling, led to salubrious changes in the immune system and better health in general. He felt that there is structuring and resolving of the harmful effects of those "hidden" feelings and images going on through the process of writing. [Pennebaker J W 1990 Opening up: the healing power of confidence in others. Avon, NY].

Danish researchers found increased natural killer cell activity among ten college students who imagined that their immune systems were becoming very effective. Natural killer cells are an important part of the immune system because they can recognize and destroy virus-infected cells, tumor cells and other invaders.

A group of metastatic cancer patients using daily imagery for a year achieved significant improvements in NK cell activity and several other measures of immune functioning.

C. Holden-Lund found that the use of an audiotape series employing relaxation with guided imagery demonstrated significantly less state anxiety, lower cortisol levels one day following surgery, and less surgical wound erythema than the control group. Thus, the guided imagery tapes demonstrated stress-relieving outcomes closely associated with healing [Res Nurs Health 1988 Aug; 11(4):235-44].

Guided Imagery Research

D.A. Rapkin, M. Straubing, and J.C. Holroyd from the University of California, Los Angeles explored the value of imagery-hypnosis on recovery from head and neck cancer surgery and found there were fewer surgical complications and less blood loss during surgery [Int J Clin Exp Hypn 1991 Oct; 39(4): 215-26].

L. LeShan found that psychological conditions had an enormous influence not only on the production of cancer, but also on the disease's evolution and even on the person's response to a particular treatment (LeShan L, Worthington R 1956 Personality as a factor in the pathogenesis of cancer: a review of the literature. British Journal of Medical Psychology 29:49-56).

K. Kolcaba and C. Fox measured the effectiveness of customized guided imagery for increasing comfort in early stage cancer. They found that listening to a guided imagery audiotape once a day for the duration of the study indicated a significant overall increase in comfort over time, and was especially salient in the first three weeks of therapy. [Oncol Nurs Forum 1999 Jan-Feb; 26(1): 67-72].

M. Jasnoski of George Washington University, Washington, D.C., is examining the effects of imagery on the immune system, with potential implications for use in cancer and AIDS.

Blair Justice of the University of Texas Health Sciences Center in Houston was funded to conduct a controlled study examining the effects of a group imagery/relaxation process on immune function and quality of life in breast cancer patients

Articles on Guided Imagery

Strategies For Implementing A Guided Imagery Program To Enhance Patient Experience
Reviews the use of and research about guided imagery in surgery, and describes how to implement a program.
2000 AACN Clin Issues 11; 1:68-76
Tusek, D. L. and Cwynar, R. E.

Imagine This! Infinite Uses Of Guided Imagery In Women's Health
Reviews use of guided imagery in outpatient, inpatient, chronic care and home care settings related to women's health.
1999 J Holist Nurs 17; 4:317-30
Bazzo, D. J. and Moeller, R. A.

The Value Of Imagery In Preoperative Nursing
Review of interactive imagery with an institutional implementation plan.
1998 Semin Perioper Nurs 7; 2:108-13
Miller, T.

Guided Imagery. A Psychoneuroimmunological Intervention In Holistic Nursing Practice. Use of guided imagery as an intervention in nursing practice, and its impact on psychoneuroimmunology.
1997 J Holist Nurs 15; 2:112-27
Giedt, J. F.

Coping, Life Attitudes, And Immune Responses To Imagery And Group Support After Breast Cancer Treatment / Richardson MA. Altern Ther Health Med 1997; 3(5): 62-70.

The Effects Of Guided Imagery On Comfort Of Women With Early Stage Breast Cancer Undergoing Radiation Therapy / Kolcaba K, Fox C. Oncol Nurs Forum 1999; 26(1): 67-72.

Imagery And Hypnosis In The Treatment Of Cancer Patients / Spiegel D. Oncology (Huntingt) 1997; 11(8): 1179-89; discussion 1189-95.

Psychological, Clinical And Pathological Effects Of Relaxation Training And Guided Imagery During Primary Chemotherapy / Walker LG, Walker MB, et al. Br J Cancer 1999; 80(1-2): 262-8.

Relaxation And Imagery For Symptom Management: Improving Patient Assessment And Individualizing Treatment / Van Fleet S. Oncol Nurs Forum 2000; 27(3): 501-10.

Use Of Relaxation For The Promotion Of Comfort And Pain Relief In Persons With Advanced Cancer / Solman R. Contemp Nurse 1994; 3(1): 6-12.

HOW TO ORDER VIDEOS, DVDS, & BOOKS

To buy any of the following Books, Videos, DVDs check with your local bookstore, or www.cancerimagery.com or email bodymindheal@aol.com, or call 949-263-4676.

VIDEOS & DVDS

Preparing Mentally & Emotionally
For Cancer Surgery
A Guided Imagery Program

Preparing Mentally Emotionally
For Cancer Chemotherapy
A Guided Imagery Program

Preparing Mentally & Emotionally
For Cancer Radiation
A Guided Imagery Program

Preparing Mentally & Emotionally
For Cancer Recovery
A Guided Imagery Program

Dissolving & Destroying Cancer Cells
A Guided Imagery Program

Pain Relief Subliminal Program
Let Your Unconscious Mind Do it!

Fear & Stress Relief Subliminal
Program Let Your Unconscious
Mind Do The Work!

30-Day Subliminal Weight Loss
Program Let Your Unconscious
Mind Do The Work!

30-Day Subliminal Stop Smoking
Program Let Your Unconscious
Mind Do The Work!

BOOKS

Cancer Guided Imagery Program
Radiation, Chemotherapy, Surgery,
And Recovery

Stop Eating Junk!
5 Minutes A Day 21-Day
Program

The Reiki Ultimate Guide
Learn Sacred Symbols and Attunements
Plus Reiki Secrets You Should Know

ABOUT THE AUTHOR

Steve Murray is a Certified Hypnotherapist and Author. He is a member of the National League of Medical Hypnotherapists and the National Guild of Hypnotists. Steve has produced a series of Cancer Guided Imagery video and DVD programs that are used in support groups and hospitals throughout the country. He also has a series of successful self-help programs on weight loss, pain, smoking, fear, and stress relief. Steve has a private practice and works with groups.

Steve can be contacted through the publisher or directly at: bodymindheal@aol.com

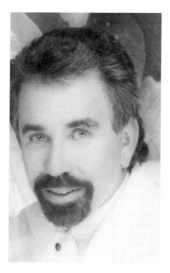